DIRECTIONS IN DEVELOPMENT

Class Action

Improving School Performance in the Developing World through Better Health and Nutrition

Joy Miller Del Rosso

Tonia Marek

The World Bank
Washington, D.C.

Joy Miller Del Rosso is with the World Bank's Human Development Department.
Tonia Marek is with the Population and Human Resources Division of the World
Bank's West Africa Department.

Cover photo: L. Goodsmith, UNICEF

Library of Congress Cataloging-in-Publication Data

Del Rosso, Joy Miller.
    Class action : improving school performance in the developing
  world through better health and nutrition / Joy Miller Del Rosso,
  Tonia Marek.
        p.   cm. — (Directions in development)
    Includes bibliographical references.
    ISBN 0-8213-3672-X
    1. Schoolchildren—Health and hygiene—Developing countries.
  2. Malnutrition in children—Developing countries.   3. Children—
  Developing countries—Nutrition.   I. Marek, Tonia.   II. Title.
  III. Series: Directions in development (Washington, D.C.)
  LB3409.D48D45   1996
  371.7'16'091724—dc20   96-9495
                                                                      CIP

Contents

Boxes

Table

Foreword

The success of survival programs for children under 5 in the developing world has created new challenges for improving the quality of life for the survivors: those who reach school age. When children are hobbled by poor nutrition and ill health, their weakened condition reduces their learning capacity and forces them to end their school careers prematurely or keeps them out of school altogether. Moreover, the ill health of this population diminishes the health and productivity of the general population and of future generations: diseases that strike children are also a source of infection for infants and adults, and when these children grow up, the wider society bears the burden of unhealthy, work-impaired adults and of the sickly and disabled infants born to them.

This book summarizes how better nutrition and health for youths will enhance:

- School enrollment, attendance, and performance
- Economic productivity
- The health of future generations.

By discussing the many low-cost and highly efficient actions that can improve school-age children's health and nutrition, this book serves as a tool for task managers to use in policy dialogue with governments, in raising consciousness and promoting interest, and in carrying out specific tasks.

Today components of about a dozen World Bank–assisted education projects address the nutrition and health of school-age children in a significant way, and additional components are in preparation. These programs—many of which have been undertaken jointly with the United Nations Children's Fund, the World Health Organization, and other partners—are new and require careful nurturing and continued support. Expansion of such programs requires stronger collaboration among donors, nongovernmental organizations, and private sector entities. The World Bank is committed to building school-based nutrition and health programs and to developing these partnerships to help ensure a brighter future for children of all ages.

David de Ferranti
Director
Human Development Department
The World Bank

1
School-Age Children at Risk

The nutrition and health of school-age children in the developing world has, until recently, received scant attention. In principle, the health sector and the education sector each offer separate avenues of approach to the problem. But in the health sector, child care focuses on pregnant women and on children through age 5. The assumption seems to be that older children have passed the critical period for child mortality and are healthier and better nourished than the very young; moreover, it was once thought that malnutrition in the preschool years permanently impairs learning capacity. Certain conditions, such as severe iodine deficiency, can indeed produce irreversible mental damage. It is now known, however, that in many cases health care and good nutrition in the school years can restore any vitality lost in the preschool years because of illness and malnutrition.

As for the education sector, the assumption that schoolchildren have passed the "survival of the fittest" test seems to have turned the attention of the education community away from students' health problems and the hurdle they represent for educational achievement. Education spending has focused instead on expanding facilities, materials, and teacher training. The nutrition and health problems of the school-age child have thus fallen through the crack between the health and education sectors.

Fortunately, this situation is beginning to change. With the gains in child survival—the proportion of children living beyond age 5 in the developing world today is almost 90 percent, versus 72 percent in 1950—the health sector has broadened its concern to the school-age population:

- Data are beginning to show that school-age children may not, in fact, be healthier than younger children.
- Clinical trials show a critical link between learning and schoolchildren's health and nutrition, suggesting a substantial potential gain in educational effectiveness from improving children's nutrition and health.
- Analyses of disease control priorities have established that school-based treatment of children is exceptionally cost-effective (see box 1). Hence, the developing world and the development community are both beginning to acknowledge the problem of health among school-age children, the importance of improving it, and the efficacy of school-based programs in doing so.

1

Box 1. The Cost-Effectiveness of School-Based Nutrition and Health Services

School-based nutrition and health services are one of the most cost-effective health interventions. Schools frequently offer social service systems that reach children more easily and provide much greater community outreach than health clinics. Children either are already at the school when treatment is offered or, if not enrolled, are brought there specifically to receive the service.

Health intervention	Cost per DALY gained (1990 U.S. dollars)
EPI Plus	12–30
School nutrition and health programs	20–34
Family planning services	20–150
Integrated management of the sick child	30–100
Prenatal and delivery care	30–100
Tobacco and alcohol prevention programs	35–55

Note: DALY, disability-adjusted life year (see chapter 2); EPI, Expanded Programme on Immunization.
Source: Bobadilla and others 1994.

Clearly, programs for improving the nutrition and health of the school-age child must not divert resources from preschool programs, which remain critically important. Nor are they a substitute for a good home environment, especially one with a high level of parental stimulation, which greatly enhances learning capacity. But no longer can the health and nutritional status of school-age children be ignored.

This book details the educational and economic gains to be had from improving the nutrition and health of the school-age population and points the way to highly cost-effective means of attaining those gains. To begin with, how severe are the health problems of the school-age child in the developing world and what are the educational gains to be had? Chapter 2 discusses what is known, with special reference to Africa.

Note

Dollars are current U.S. dollars, unless otherwise specified. A billion is 1,000 million.

2
Costly Conditions, Low-Cost Remedies

Many nutrition and health problems afflicting preschool children—malaria, immunizable childhood diseases, respiratory infections, diarrheal diseases, protein and energy malnutrition, and vitamin and mineral deficiencies—persist through the school years. Moreover, some maladies, such as parasitic diseases, tuberculosis, and anemia—the latter particularly in girls following puberty—may become more prevalent and intense during the school years.

Nutritional and health status are powerful influences on a child's learning capacity and on how well that child performs in school. Children who lack certain nutrients in their diet (particularly iron and iodine), or who suffer from protein-energy malnutrition, hunger, and parasitic infections or other diseases, do not have the same capacity for learning as healthy and well-nourished children. Weak health and poor nutrition among school-age children diminish their cognitive development either through physiological changes or by reducing their ability to participate in learning experiences—or both.

Curing Infectious and Parasitic Diseases

A starting point for examining the health and nutrition problems of school-age children is the recent work on the burden of disease in Sub-Saharan Africa (see table 1). The disease burden is measured in disability-adjusted life years (DALYs), which combine healthy life years lost because of premature mortality with years lost as a result of disability. The leading cause of illness and death among children from birth through age 4—as well as for the age group 5 through 14—is communicable diseases. Malnutrition increases children's susceptibility to most of these communicable diseases and also increases the severity of the disease.

Malaria

Among communicable illnesses, malaria is the greatest disabler of both younger children and the school-aged.[1] School-age children in malarial

Table 1. DALYs Lost because of Major Communicable Diseases,
Sub-Saharan Africa, Estimates for 1990
(percentage of total loss)

Disease	Age (years)	
	5–14	0–4
Malaria	12.9	15.1
Childhood cluster	12.6	14.9
Measles	7.0	8.6
Tropical cluster	9.7	0.3
Schistosomiasis	6.7	0.1
Diarrheal diseases	7.8	17.0
Respiratory infections	7.8	16.5
Tuberculosis	6.7	0.5
Intestinal worms	2.2	0.0

Note: DALY, disability-adjusted life year.
Source: Murray and Lopez 1994.

areas are thought to have acquired a natural immunity to the disease
through repeated exposure at a younger age, but in reality two factors,
seasonality and urbanization, delay the onset of this natural immunity.
In some regions, such as the Sahel, malaria is seasonal, and the reduc-
tion of infection in the off-season slows the acquisition of immunity.
Likewise, an urbanized area, with fewer habitats for mosquitoes, reduces the incidence of malaria in young children, leaving them more
susceptible to infection in their school-age years.

In addition, two disabling conditions—tuberculosis and infection by
helminths (parasitic worms)—are much more prevalent among school-
agers than among young children. Currently, the schools have no
obvious role in addressing tuberculosis, but they can help in the fight
against helminths.[2]

Helminths: Intestinal Worms and Schistosomes

Parasitic worms that infect the intestines or the blood are a major source
of disease and malnutrition in school-age children. Intestinal worms
known as roundworm (*Ascaris*), whipworm (*Trichuris*), and hookworm
(*Necator* and *Ancylostoma*) are the most prevalent of the more than thirty
helminths that can infect humans. An estimated 400 million school-age
children are infected with roundworm, 300 million with whipworm, and
170 million with hookworm.

Schistosomiasis, the presence in the blood of the parasitic schistosome
worm, affects an estimated 200 million people throughout the world,
approximately 88 million of whom are under 15 years old. Ninety percent

of all schistosomiasis is found in Africa (WHO 1995). In highly endemic areas three of four children may be infected; the consequent disease burden (loss of DALYs) for males age 5 to 14 is second only to that from malaria.[3]

THE CONSEQUENCES OF PARASITIC INFECTIONS. Parasitic infections in children can produce malnutrition, diarrhea, anorexia, and general malaise. Children heavily infected with worms eat less, even when food is available, and their absorption and retention of certain nutrients is impaired. The malnutrition attendant on parasitic infection diminishes children's learning capacity and their ability to pay attention and concentrate. Research shows that even when infections seem to produce no overt symptoms (diarrhea, abdominal pain, and so on), they can diminish growth and cognitive development (Nokes and others 1992a).

THE BENEFITS OF TREATING PARASITIC INFECTIONS IN SCHOOL-AGE CHILDREN. Ridding children of worms allows them to eat more, absorb more, and hence lose less food value from their diet. Twice the normal growth rate has been observed in stunted children after drug treatment, even without improving their diet (Stephenson and others 1989). Treating children for intestinal helminths has also improved learning capacity. A study in Jamaica of children age 9 through 12 found that nine weeks after their treatment for worms, they scored significantly better on cognitive tests than the control group that took placebos and remained infected. On completion of the study, the treated group and the control group that was uninfected did not differ significantly in their performance on tests (Nokes and others 1992b). A single treatment of children in the West Indies for whipworm infection, without nutritional supplements or improvements in education, improved the children's learning capacity to the point that their test scores matched those of children who were uninfected (Bundy and others 1990).

Reducing Malnutrition and Hunger

Contrary to conventional wisdom, nutritional status does not improve with age.[4] The extra demands on school-age children (to perform chores, for example, or walk long distances to school) create a need for energy that is much greater than that of younger children; the school-aged, therefore, can be at higher risk for malnutrition and hunger than their siblings age 3 to 5. Indeed, the available data indicate high levels of protein-energy malnutrition and short-term hunger among school-age children. Moreover, deficiencies of such critical nutrients as iodine, vitamin A, and iron among the school-aged are pervasive. It is estimated that 60 million school-age children suffer from iodine deficiency disorders and that another 85 million are at higher risk for acute respiratory disease and other infections because they are deficient in vitamin A. The number suffering from iron deficiency anemia is greater still—210 million (Jamison and others 1993).

The High Cost of Malnourishment, the Low Cost of Remediation

Deficiencies of iron, iodine, and vitamin A are among the most destructive types of malnutrition. The human body, however, requires only minute quantities of these "micronutrients," and a number of extremely cost-effective strategies are available to supply them either pharmaceutically or through the fortification of basic foodstuffs (World Bank 1994).

IRON. Low iron is a sizable problem for all ages and is considered to be the most common nutritional deficiency in developing countries. Pregnant women, infants, and preschool children are at the greatest risk for the worst effects of iron deficiency—mental retardation or death.

Iron deficiency among the school-aged also takes a toll: it renders them listless, inattentive, and uninterested in learning. These effects are, however, reversible. In India iron supplementation virtually eliminated the differences in school performance and IQ scores between schoolchildren previously deficient in iron and those without iron deficiencies (Seshadri and Gopaldas 1989). When the diets of children in Malawi were supplemented with iron as well as iodine, the gain in IQ scores was even greater than with iodine alone (Shrestha 1994). Iron deficiency also reduces resistance to infection and possibly inhibits growth; some studies of school-age children have found that alleviation of iron deficiency is associated with weight gain (Chwang, Soemantri, and Pollitt 1988).

IODINE. If a pregnant woman suffers from serious iodine deficiency, her newborn is much more likely than the average infant to suffer from mental retardation, poor growth, and deafness. Children who lack iodine remain at risk for further detrimental effects on learning capacity.[5] If children suffering from these ailments enter school at all, they are likely to enter late, to have more difficulty learning, and to leave prematurely.

Fortunately, inexpensive remediation is possible. Providing iodine supplementation to school-age children in an area of Bolivia with high iodine deficiency decreased the size of their goiters while improving their IQ scores, especially among girls (Bautista and others 1982). Children in Malawi who received iodine supplements had significantly increased IQs—21 points, on average (Shrestha 1994). Giving iodine supplementation to hearing-impaired, iodine-deficient children in China improved their hearing (Yan-you and Shu-hua 1985).

VITAMIN A. Deficiencies of vitamin A are most destructive in the first 5 years of life, when they can permanently blind the child. Vitamin A deficiency in school-aged children also warrants treatment. Vitamin A plays a role in immune function throughout life, and its deficiency in children has been associated with both anemia and poor growth.

In Thailand when the diets of children up to age 9 were supplemented with vitamin A, their iron stores and resistance to infection improved (Bloem and others 1990). Also, recent evidence suggests that female adolescents have a special need for vitamin A, that vitamin A may reduce anemia, and that it may reduce the vertical (mother-to-child) transmission of HIV and possibly other infections (Brabin and Brabin 1992).

Protein-Energy Malnutrition: A Risk Factor for Impaired Learning

Children with protein-energy malnutrition (PEM)—an insufficient intake of protein and energy that often interacts with infectious disease—are at risk for impaired learning capacity and poor school performance. The results of at least fifteen studies from the developing world and the United States confirm that chronic PEM in the past (as indicated by low height for age) and in the present (as indicated by low weight for height) diminishes cognitive development. PEM usually occurs in conjunction with such social and environmental conditions as poverty and lack of parental stimulation, which also contribute to impaired cognition. Research suggests, however, that PEM independently impairs learning capacity.[6]

The detrimental effects of PEM on cognitive development, like those of micronutrient deficiency, can be reversed. Even while continuing to live in an inadequate environment, children whose food intake improves demonstrate enhanced learning capacity.[7] A study in Guatemala that followed children from infancy to adolescence found that those who had received a protein supplement as young children had better achievement test scores than matched children who had received a placebo supplement (Pollitt and others 1993). A study in Jamaica, in which the intervention was a program of psychosocial stimulation for severely malnourished children, found similar benefits: fourteen years later, youngsters who had received the stimulation during early childhood had higher IQ scores and better school achievement than malnourished children in a control group who did not participate in the program. The entire group of malnourished children, however, still had markedly lower scores than the well-nourished control group (Grantham-McGregor 1993).

Hunger

The evidence that school-age children can benefit from intervention comes primarily from cross-sectional studies within ongoing programs, particularly school feeding programs. Simply alleviating hunger in schoolchildren helps them perform better in school. In Jamaica providing breakfast to primary school students significantly increased their attendance and arithmetic scores. The children who benefited most were those who were wasted, stunted, or previously malnourished (Simeon and Grantham-McGregor 1989).[8]

A U.S. study also shows the benefit of providing breakfast to disadvantaged primary school students. Before the start of a school breakfast program, eligible (low-income) children scored significantly lower on achievement tests than those not eligible. Once in the program, however, the test scores of the children participating in the program improved more than those of nonparticipants. The attendance of participating children also improved (Meyers, Sampson, and Weitzman 1989).

Studies in Benin, Burkina Faso, and Togo of the determinants of achievement found that a school meal was related to children's performance on year-end tests. In Benin, children in schools with canteens scored 5 points higher on second-grade tests than did children in schools without canteens. Of the inputs studied, only "books in the classroom" had a greater positive effect on achievement (Jarousse and Mingat 1991).

Stronger evidence of the beneficial effect of alleviating hunger in schoolchildren comes from a recent study of a school breakfast program in Peru. After only one month, children participating in the program consumed 25 percent more calories, 28 percent more protein, and 46 percent more iron than nonparticipating children and had better attendance. In a subsample of these children, scores on cognitive tests also improved (Jacoby, Cueto, and Pollitt n.d.).

Little support exists in research results or in developmental theory for the notion that malnutrition among the school-aged degrades their basic aptitudes (whereas support does exist for that notion in regard to infancy and early childhood). But PEM and hunger during the school years does affect, at a minimum, attention and concentration—and probably other factors that also influence learning, absenteeism, and duration of schooling.

Notes

1. The cluster of childhood diseases comprising pertussis, poliomyelitis, diphtheria, measles, and tetanus comes in a close second to malaria for both age groups. Respiratory infections and diarrheal diseases also are widespread in both groups. Childhood immunizable diseases afflict the entire age spectrum of children in African countries because these countries have the lowest rates of immunization worldwide. Schools have a role to play in promoting and delivering immunizations, but children under age 5 remain the target group for intervention.

2. Tuberculosis is curable in a clinical setting through either short-course or standard-course chemotherapy; the short course uses three to five drugs over a six-to-eight-month period, and the standard course uses two to three drugs over a twelve-to-eighteen-month period. In all chemotherapy scenarios the cost of treatment is less than $10 per DALY gained. The vaccine BCG should be given at birth to prevent tuberculosis through age 14. Some authorities recommend a second treatment of BCG at the time children begin or end their schooling. (The drug's effectiveness in adults remains controversial.) More attention to tuberculosis treatment and prevention is warranted because of the magnitude of the problem and because it has been ignored in the international health community for the past fifteen years.

3. The schistosome worm is carried by several species of water-associated snails that can pass the worm to adults and children who use or play in snail-infested waters.

4. The assumption in this regard with respect to Zimbabwe, for example, was that levels of undernutrition in the preschool years declined to more acceptable levels in school-age children. Early data collected in schools seemed to show an improvement. Now, however, it is recognized that the data probably reflected the higher dropout rates among malnourished children. More recent data collected on all age groups in one region show that children age 6 through 10 had similar levels of stunting (low height for age) and more wasting (low weight for height) than children age 2 through 5 (Tagwireyi and Greiner 1994). During the 1984 drought in Kenya, food intake among school-age children declined, while that of preschoolers remained constant (McDonald and others 1994).

5. In Sicily, for example, the proportion of children with below-normal cognitive scores was 3 percent in areas with sufficient iodine, 18.5 percent in areas where iodine was inadequate, and 19.3 percent in areas where iodine was inadequate and cretinism was endemic (Vermiglio and others 1990). Studies in Indonesia and Spain have documented similar effects on children in areas with insufficient iodine (Bleichrodt, Drenth, and Querido 1980; Bleichrodt and others 1987).

6. In Thailand a study of more than 2,000 children found that after removing the effects of social and environmental factors, variables indicative of nutritional status (head circumference and height for age) predicted school achievement scores (Kotchabhakdi and others 1989). In the Philippines children of normal nutritional status outperformed children with poor nutritional status, even when family income, school quality, and teacher's ability were taken into account

(Florencio 1987). Similarly, in Kenya researchers linked actual food intake with cognitive and educational measures after controlling for socioeconomic factors. Children who were better nourished had higher scores on tests of verbal comprehension and IQ (Sigman and others 1989).

7. All of the research projects that examined the potential to overcome the detrimental effects of PEM over time have targeted preschool children. This targeting, which reflects the nutrition and health community's focus on children under age 5, acknowledges that in compensating children for deficits, the earlier the intervention the better.

8. Even temporary hunger, common among children who are not fed before going to school, can have an adverse effect on learning. Children who are hungry have more difficulty concentrating and performing complex tasks, even if they are otherwise well nourished. In Canada a study of the effect of missing breakfast (short-term hunger) among low-income children found that "low-achieving" children ate breakfast less regularly than did "high-performing" children from similar home environments (Houde-Nadeau and Hunter n.d.). In Africa the detrimental effects of hunger on learning are exacerbated by malnutrition.

3
Higher Productivity and Better Community Health

A community's educational and economic status is closely linked to its health status: improve its nutrition and health and its education and economy will be strengthened. Addressing nutrition and health among the school-aged does more than improve the health and learning capacity of the treatment group—benefits detailed in the preceding chapter. It brings intergenerational nutrition and health benefits and long-term economic gains as well. The lesson of this book is that bettering nutrition and health among the school-aged, like the critical effort to improve nutrition and health among infants, is a strategic element in the effort to develop the community:

- Healthier and better nourished children stay in school longer, learn more, and become healthier and more productive adults.
- Girls who stay in school longer tend to delay childbearing longer than school-leavers, and merely delaying childbearing brings the intergenerational benefits of a lowered birth rate, better birth outcomes, and better child health.
- School-age children with lower levels of disease reduce the overall transmission of disease in the wider community.

Only by considering these broader, longer-term benefits can one have a sense of the total return from investing in the nutrition and health of school-age children.

Raising School Attendance and Performance

Poor nutrition and health among schoolchildren contribute to the inefficiency of the educational system. Children with diminished cognitive abilities and sensory impairments naturally perform less well and are more likely to repeat grades and to drop out of school than children who are not impaired; they also enroll in school at a later age, if at all, and finish fewer years of schooling. The irregular school attendance of malnourished and unhealthy children is one of the key factors in their poor performance. Research and program experience show that

11

improving nutrition and health can lead to better performance, fewer repeated grades, and less dropping out. School-based nutrition and health programs can also motivate parents to enroll their children in school and to see that they attend regularly.

Improving Enrollment

Children in poor health start school later in life or not at all. A study in Nepal found that the probability of attending school was 5 percent for stunted children versus 27 percent for children of normal nutritional status (Moock and Leslie 1986). In Ghana malnourished children entered school at a later age and completed fewer years of school than better nourished children (Glewwe and Jacoby 1994).

The number of days that a child attends school is related to cognition and performance (Ceci 1995; Jacoby, Cueto, and Pollitt n.d.). School feeding programs, by far the most common nutrition intervention aimed at school-age children and the one with the largest monetary benefit to families, have a positive effect on rates of enrollment and attendance.

A recent evaluation of a school feeding program in Burkina Faso found that school canteens were associated with increased school enrollment, regular attendance, consistently lower repeater rates, lower dropout rates in the more disadvantaged provinces, and higher success rates on national exams, especially among girls (Moore 1994). In the Dominican Republic up to 25 percent of children dropped out of school during a period without a school feeding program; the effect was greatest in rural areas and for girls (King 1990). School enrollment in Honduras increased 12 percent following the distribution of food stamps in schools, and repetition and dropout rates declined (World Bank 1992).

Improving Achievement

A large-scale study in China showed that a child's height for age predicted grade level. For each standard-deviation increase in height in relationship to age, the child was 0.3 year further ahead in school (Jamison 1985). Similarly, in Nepal height for age predicted grade attainment (Moock and Leslie 1986).

A study over many years in Guatemala found consistently better past nutrition (greater height for age) and current nutrition (greater weight for height) associated with higher cognitive test scores and better school performance (Pollitt and others 1993). In Honduras stunted children (smaller height for age) who came from the poorest homes were twice as likely to repeat a grade as were nonstunted children from such homes (Israel, Wilson, and Praun n.d.). In northeastern Brazil the school achievement of malnourished children was 20 percent behind that of children with normal nutritional status and vision, and the school achievement of those with poor eyesight was 27 percent behind. Both impaired groups experienced below-average school promotion and above-average dropout rates (Harbison and Hanushek 1992).

Improving Nutrition and Health, Now and in the Future

The benefits to the whole community from alleviating poor nutrition and improving health in school-age children have up to now been little appreciated, in large part because the assumption about the health of the school-aged has been too optimistic. We can only estimate the poor state of health and nutrition among the school-aged, but we do know that school-age children suffer significantly from many of the same diseases and injuries as younger children, and in some places their burden may be even greater.

The complete health picture of school-age children is not, however, reflected in the data. DALYs lost to conditions such as malnutrition, which have their onset in infancy, are attributed to the burden of illness in children under 5 years old, yet part of this burden will be felt during the school-age years. So treating the school-age population will confer a significant benefit not only on the school-agers themselves, but also—at present and as they grow older—on future generations.

Benefiting the Wider Community

The treatment of diseases prevalent in the school-age population weakens a major source of community infection. The results can be dramatic. In the Caribbean island of Montserrat, for example, more than 90 percent of schoolchildren age 4 through 12 were treated at four-month intervals for two and one-half years with an anthelmintic (antiworm) drug. Less than 4 percent of adults received treatment during the same period. As expected, the incidence of parasitic infection in the school population declined to almost zero. But infections in the adult population declined an almost equal amount because of reduced transmission from the school-age population (Bundy and others 1990).

Benefiting the Current School-Age Population as It Ages

Health-related behaviors developed during school age influence the risk of developing subsequent illness. School age extends well beyond age 14, the cutoff for "childhood"; it encompasses childhood through adolescence and early adulthood. Therefore, not only are childhood diseases a concern; so too are adolescent and adult health issues. Experiencing better health, learning about nutrition and the avoidance of disease, and, for older school-agers, learning to avoid sexually transmitted disease all serve the school-aged—and those around them—throughout their lives.

Benefiting Future Generations

Girls, particularly adolescent girls, are the key to the health of future generations. Good physiological development during adolescence prepares girls for pregnancy, childbirth, and motherhood. Ensuring that girls are well nourished and healthy—especially regarding their increased needs for iron and for growth before the reproductive years begin—will decrease the incidence of low birth weight and birth defects in their children and will reduce their risk of dying during childbirth.

Adolescence is also the age at which young people begin to make independent decisions about their health and to form attitudes and adopt behaviors that influence their current and future health as well as the health of their future children. Schools may offer one of the best venues for providing adolescent girls with critical nutrition and health services and for reaching all young people with the information and education that will help them lead healthier lives. In Tamil Nadu, for example, a school feeding program attracted more girls to attend school and improved the attendance of those already in school. In addition to benefiting educationally, these girls had the opportunity to learn about family planning. As a result they had fewer children when they reached child-bearing age (Devadas 1983).[1]

In most African countries the school enrollment of girls lags significantly behind that of boys. Addressing this gender issue is critical to increasing school enrollment and reaping the intergenerational health gains to be had from healthier, better-informed, teenage girls. Because they can have a greater effect on girls than on boys, nutrition and health interventions could help close the gender gap in school enrollment. Girls, for example, suffer more than boys from deficiencies of iron and iodine. The study in Bolivia discussed previously found that the positive effect on IQ scores of reducing goiter was greater among school-age girls than among school-age boys (Bautista and others 1982).

School feeding programs can also improve the enrollment rate of girls relative to boys, as was shown by a large-scale evaluation of such a program in India (Gupta and Hom 1984). Moreover, some school feeding programs have been explicitly designed to have a disproportionate effect on the school enrollment of girls; a program in Ghana achieves that goal by giving the girls a take-home ration in addition to the meal at school (Catholic Relief Services 1993a). A similar approach has been effectively used in Pakistan and the Republic of Yemen (UNESCO n.d.).

Note

1. Studies in the United States have shown that health education programs are cost-effective. Every $1 invested in education on the hazards of tobacco use saves an estimated $18.80 in the costs required to address the problems associated with smoking. A $1 investment in programs aimed at the prevention of drug and alcohol abuse yields savings of $5.69. A $1 investment in education to prevent unprotected sexual behavior saves $5.10 (Rothman and Collins forthcoming).

4
Taking Action

With attention only recently turned to the health and nutrition needs of the school-age population, experience with programs is still relatively limited, particularly in Africa, where the survival of children under 5 years remains a significant problem. Nevertheless, enough is known from experience in other parts of the world to recommend actions. Many illnesses that affect the school-aged can be treated effectively and safely, most with inexpensive methods. And even those conditions whose treatment costs are higher (for example, hunger) are worth treating.

The goal is to establish broad-based programs of health and nutrition for the school-aged using what is already known. Almost all countries have some knowledge of the health problems that affect the school-aged, and some already have an agency responsible for school-based nutrition and health programs. But in many cases that agency has no funding or offers only one specific service, such as a feeding program. The strategy we chart here toward a thriving school-age population harnesses political commitment and the support of local and international donors while deploying the most effective and affordable health and nutrition interventions.

The tactics of this approach encompass (a) a rapid, low-cost assessment of the health and nutrition of the school-aged to identify high-priority targets for intervention and to galvanize governmental and donor support, (b) appropriate low-cost, high-return interventions, as indicated by the assessment, (c) targeting of school feeding programs to enhance their cost-effectiveness, (d) a longer-term program to improve the physical school environment so that school health and nutrition services are supported, and (e) education to change behaviors related to health, nutrition, and hygiene.

Analyzing the Situation

Engaging governments in a national situation analysis is one of the best ways to heighten their awareness of the needs of school-age children. An analysis of existing information and, if needed, a rapid assessment in the field keep governments focused and energized and avoid a protracted, expensive, and perhaps bureaucratically complex study; instead, governments can quickly grasp the problem and launch a discussion of solutions. Several donor agencies and governments have supported such analyses.

A recent assessment in Malawi, for example, exposed the gravity of the nutritional and health situation of school-age children and formed the basis for a national planning workshop on school-based nutrition and health interventions. The workshop led to recommendations for a series of short-term interventions to meet the most immediate nutrition and health needs, including deworming, micronutrient distribution, and information and education programs. A basic education project, supported by the World Bank, is being prepared to assist the Malawians in taking the next steps to address these priority needs.

Conducting a Situation Analysis

The objective of a situation analysis is to guide the design and development of programing. Governments need information on the health status of school-age children, on school attendance (enrollment, absentee, and dropout rates), and on existing school nutrition and health programs. Considerations of age and gender and of seasonal, geographic, and other patterns are important. A significant aspect of a situation analysis is that it builds relationships among the actors responsible for using the information gathered and between these actors and the communities they must address.

The appropriate method of collecting information will vary by needs, circumstances, and resources; techniques include collecting routine statistics, making special surveys, conducting interviews, and holding focus group discussions with students, parents, teachers, and health workers. The Partnership for Child Development has developed a protocol for a comprehensive situation analysis of school-based nutrition and health interventions, which is being tested in several African countries (see appendix A). It constitutes a menu of approaches, from which countries can choose to satisfy their specific needs and still stay within their resources.

Targeting via a Census

A tool for identifying target groups that is widely used in Latin America and Eastern Europe is a census that records the height and age of first-grade children. The growth of children in underprivileged populations is determined mainly by environmental factors such as food intake and illness. The height-for-age census, therefore, can quickly identify needy geographic areas. It can also be used for planning, programming, evaluation, and advocacy. It obtains these rich results at low cost—about 10 cents per child—and can be implemented within a few months. The census can also provide an updated register of schools, including the number of first-grade children and their age at entry.

The census technique may be less valuable for targeting programs in countries where malnourishment is widespread; nonetheless, almost all countries have some potential for targeting. National surveys of other specific conditions can also identify high-risk areas quickly and cheaply. A national parasite incidence survey in Guinea cost approximately $30,000 and was implemented within three months.

Three Cost-Effective Nutrition and Health Interventions

Three school-based nutrition and health interventions in use today are relatively easy to deliver, low in cost, and highly effective in ameliorating high-priority nutrition and health problems: (a) mass application of anthelmintics (deworming medications), (b) delivery of micronutrients, particularly iron and iodine, and (c) treatment of injuries and routine health problems along with classroom management of students' sensory deficits (impaired hearing and vision).

These three programs are low in cost because they generally can be delivered by schoolteachers with only minimal participation by health personnel. Certain situations may warrant the modification of these basic strategies: for example, where enrollments are low, efforts to serve

---

Box 2. Reaching Out-of-School Children

The proportion of eligible girls enrolled in primary school in Guinea is about 30 percent nationwide. Thus, school-based health interventions—treatment for worms, iodine supplementation, and health education—have been designed to reach not only students but out-of-school children as well, especially girls of child-bearing age. The program, currently being implemented on a trial basis in several areas, is run by school parent-teacher associations, which include a head teacher in collaboration with community health extension agents. The parents collect money from the community and order and pick up drugs and micronutrients. Over time, parent-teacher associations will also develop and implement the social marketing communications program. Initial results indicate that this community-based approach is effective in reaching enrolled and nonenrolled children, the latter making up more than 50 percent of the children treated in trial areas.

> **Box 3. The Right Drug**
>
> Broad-spectrum, single-dose drugs effective against several species of worm are now available to treat intestinal helminths. Albendazole (400-milligram single dose) and Mebendazole (500-milligram single dose) are both nearly 100 percent effective in eradicating roundworm (*Ascaris*) infection. As for hookworm (*Necator* and *Ancylostoma*), mean egg counts are reduced 98 percent by Albendazole and 82 percent by Mebendazole. Neither drug is effective in clearing whipworm (*Trichuris*), but both reduce egg counts by about 70 percent, enough to markedly reduce the incidence of disease arising from the infection. Praziquantel (40-milligram per kilogram of body weight, single dose) is effective against all forms of schistosomiasis.
>
> Choosing a drug depends on cost, safety, and efficacy. The cost differential between Albendazole and Mebendazole is significant: 20 cents per dose for Albendazole, 3 cents per dose for Mebendazole. Praziquantel has cost about 50 cents per treatment, although the major producer recently cut its price to 30 cents. Other producers are also likely to reduce prices.
>
> Ensuring drug quality is critical. Governments have reportedly purchased drugs for school programs that proved to be ineffective when tested (personal communication, Donald Bundy). Only certain distributors provide effective drugs; a list of these distributors is available through UNICEF.

children who are not enrolled and children who are enrolled but who do not attend (absentees) are necessary; see box 2. But these changes may not necessarily increase the cost of intervention.

Helminth Control

School-based helminth control delivers deworming drugs to children through their schools without first testing for infection. Remedies are inexpensive (see box 3), easy to deliver, and thus highly cost-effective. Bypassing diagnosis not only decreases cost but also increases compliance by the children because of peer relations ("we all take the medicine, so I am not different from anyone else when I take it") and because some children would not submit to the diagnosis procedure, which requires the collection of a stool sample. Moreover, because school-age children typically harbor the most intense helminth infections, treatment of this group, as noted in the previous chapter, is one of the best ways to reduce infection in the entire community.

TARGETING TREATMENT. The communities to receive mass deworming treatment through the schools are carefully targeted on the basis of risk of disease. Communities with a large proportion of people infected (usually more than 50 percent) also have the highest level of illness from helminth infection. Thus, school-based treatment without screening should be implemented in areas where surveys of school-age children indicate a prevalence of intestinal helminth or schistosome infection of more than 50 percent. Treatment at prevalence rates below 50 percent may be justified in areas where multiple infections increase morbidity, or where more than 25 percent of children are malnourished, or where sanitation is particularly inadequate (WHO 1990).

BENEFITS OF TREATMENT. Although reinfection may be inevitable, drug therapy can keep worm infestation low for months or years before it builds up again to disease-producing levels. The rate of reinfection following treatment depends on the species of helminth and the local intensity of infection.

Current estimates are that treatment is required once or twice a year for roundworm (*Ascaris*) and whipworm (*Trichuris*) and every two years for hookworm (*Necator* and *Ancylostoma*) to achieve acceptable levels of reinfection. These intervals assume coverage of 80–90 percent of the targeted school-age population; if coverage is substantially lower, reinfection will occur more quickly. For schistosomiasis, the treatment interval (time between treatments) is much longer—from two to five years, depending on level of transmission.

Alleviating Micronutrient Deficiencies

As with school-based helminth control programs, school-based micro-nutrient supplementation programs are based on the premise that a large proportion of school-age children are appropriate targets and that treatment can be delivered at school. Indeed, a large proportion of children are deficient in certain micronutrients, especially iron, iodine, and vitamin A, and supplements are easily and inexpensively delivered in a school setting. The provision of a 100–200-milligram ferrous sulfate tablet once a week to school-age children is being tested for its efficacy in ameliorating iron deficiency. Such a regimen is less time-consuming than the standard clinical treatment of a daily tablet.

A 400–960-milligram capsule of iodized oil once a year alleviates iodine deficiency in children age 6 to 15 and in women of childbearing age. To alleviate vitamin A deficiency, a 200,000-IU (international unit) capsule every four to six months is effective.

COSTS OF SUPPLEMENTATION. The costs of micronutrients are quite low: vitamin A capsules cost 2 cents a dose, and only two or three doses a year are required; a single annual dose of iodine costs 32 cents; and at one tablet per school week, a year's worth of iron folate tablets costs less than 10 cents a child. These costs exclude shipping, handling, and internal local delivery costs (UNICEF 1995).

Few data from large-scale operational programs are available, but by using readily available channels—for example, piggybacking on essential drug programs—and by using the school infrastructure and personnel at the district and local levels (for obtaining supplies) and teachers (for administration), costs can presumably be kept low. In the state of Gujarat in India, for example, 3 million primary school students receive a midday meal. To improve the value of this program, a package including vitamin A, an iron supplement, and the antiworm drug Albendazole is provided to students along with the meal at no additional cost to the school system. The training and delivery involved in this program uses the existing infrastructure, and local manufacturers of the drug and the supplements absorb the costs of delivery to the district level (Gopaldas and Gujral 1996).

SCHOOL PROGRAMS AND NATIONWIDE STRATEGY. School programs can be used in the interim while more general programs take shape and also to cover areas missed by national efforts. Fortification—the addition of specific vitamins and minerals to foods and water—is a general program for alleviating micronutrient deficiencies. National programs to fortify salt with iodine are in various stages of development in most African countries, but many areas with moderate to severe iodine deficiency will not be adequately covered within an acceptable period of time. As an interim measure, supplementation with iodized oil capsules is recommended, and such programs can be school based. Similarly, once fortification programs are fully launched, school-based supplementation programs for iron, iodine, and vitamin A can be concentrated in areas still not covered by national programs.

FORTIFIED FOODS. The fortification of a school meal or snack can also meet micronutrient needs. An urban school feeding program in the Dominican Republic, for example, fortifies the program's bread ration with 100 percent of the daily iron requirement (see box 4). A similar program in Peru uses fortified foods in the school breakfast program to deliver 100 percent of the iron requirement and 60 percent of the requirements of other micronutrients in the school breakfast. The World Food Program now includes iodized salt in its school feeding programs.

Box 4. Fortified Breakfast: A Low-Cost Intervention for Iron Deficiency

A simple approach to alleviating iron deficiency in schoolchildren is under way in the Dominican Republic. A special cornmeal fortified with 100 percent of the recommended daily intake of iron for children from 6 years through 10 years is part of the recipe for the muffins and cookies provided to poor urban schoolchildren. All suppliers purchase the fortified cornmeal directly from the one corn mill in the country. The equipment to mix the iron into the cornmeal cost $3,000 (1996 dollars); the cost of the iron itself is 3 cents a child per year. The fortified cornmeal product will also be incorporated into the breakfast porridge provided to rural schoolchildren.

Addressing Other Health Problems

Given their much wider access to children when compared to health clinics, schools can be a more efficient way to deliver some aspects of primary health care to children. Such efforts have seen some success in the United States (see box 5) and may be feasible and appropriate for some parts of the developing world. Schools in most developing regions, however, are not likely to be in a position to establish a comprehensive school-based clinical health program. Even so, many simple health treatments with high benefits do not require medical supervision. Providing schools with a medicine kit costs little and yet can address some of the

---

Box 5. School-Based Health Clinics: The U.S. Experience

One of the United States' first school-based clinics, available to the child from birth through high school in the Boston-area city of Cambridge, Massachusetts, helped put local immunization levels at 98 percent, compared with the national average of 60 percent; reduced the proportion of children with elevated levels of lead in their blood from 7 percent to 0.5 percent; reduced the incidence of anemia from 16 percent to 4 percent; and reduced the inappropriate use of hospital emergency rooms by half.

This experience and others have established the following prerequisites for effective programs: (a) the school must have at least 1,000 students for the clinic to be cost-effective, (b) the facility must be on or near the school grounds, (c) a variety of health professionals must be on the staff, (d) funding must come predominantly from the health establishment, not from the educational budget, (e) the clinic must offer comprehensive services, from diagnosis and treatment to counseling, and (f) the clinic must be linked to the larger health care network. (See Butler and Porter 1994.)

Box 6. Malaria Control through Insecticide-Treated Bed Nets

The use of insecticide-treated bed nets can be an effective means for malaria control. Programs advocating their use are aimed at having a treated bed net in every household, having families use bed nets regularly and properly, and having the community re-treat the bed nets at least once each year. Social marketing provides the framework and the tools to develop a program to meet those objectives. The first steps involve consultation with the targeted community groups followed by the groups' participation in formulating and testing products. The consultation and testing give program planners the information they need to decide on the bed net itself, its cost, the scope of the market, the mechanisms for delivering the product, and a communications strategy, all focused on inducing a practice that does not now exist—the widespread and effective use of bed nets. (See Griffiths and Favin 1993.)

---

most chronic health problems of school-age children.[1] The timely treatment of a small wound, for instance, can prevent a more serious infection and the cost associated with it.

MALARIA. The concept of treating malaria through school-based intervention is sound, but experience with the approach is limited, and controls need to be emphasized. The indiscriminate use of antimalarial drugs has contributed to the development of drug resistance in many countries, so populations with chloroquine-resistant strains of malaria should be treated with a different drug. Chloroquine should be dispensed through schools to treat only those fevers considered to be malaria induced.[2] Seasonal criteria—such as treatment after the rainy season, when malaria prevalence is high—could also be applied. Another approach to prevention that offers much potential is using the schools to encourage the use of insecticide-impregnated bed nets (see box 6).

SENSORY-IMPAIRED CHILDREN. Poor vision and hearing among school-age children are important problems with potentially simple remedies. A situation analysis can identify the extent of this problem in the school-age population, and if it is found to be significant, teachers can be trained in the use of simple eye charts and "whisper" tests to assess their students. Sensory-impaired children might be given corrective lenses or hearing aids. If this is not feasible, teachers need to be encouraged to move these children to the front of the class or to take such helpful measures as writing larger and speaking louder. Training in these screening and classroom management techniques could be integrated with other in-service teacher training programs.

Box 7. The Cost of School Feeding Programs

A comparison of the costs of school feeding programs is problematic. The number of days of feeding varies, as does the quantity of the rations and their quality. When cross-country cost information is standardized by controlling for some of these differences, the data show that the cost of school feeding programs ranges from $19.25 to $208.59 per 1,000 calories per student per day for 365 days (1989 dollars). The mean program cost was $88.74, the median $81.46. These costs are comparable to those of other types of feeding programs. (See Horton 1992.)

Reducing Hunger

Alleviating hunger in school-age children, typically by providing meals or snacks at school, is more expensive and complicated than some other school-based health and nutrition interventions. For example, food is much more costly than micronutrient supplements or anthelmintic drugs (see box 7), and the logistics of food delivery and meal preparation can be complex. Moreover, school feeding programs have a significant political dimension because they are highly visible and can represent a considerable income transfer. Nonetheless, when children go to school hungry and do not have money to buy food at school, a feeding program may be necessary if they are to take full educational advantage of being in school.[3] Reconciling the political, nutritional, financial, and logistical dimensions of school feeding programs is critical for improving current programs or developing new ones.

The problems with school feeding programs are well known:

- Food supplies—and hence, programs—tend to be irregular.
- Food is often lost, either to spoilage or to the black market.
- The rations are inadequate in calories and other nutrients.
- Money is too scarce to offer a daily ration.
- The food is unpalatable or unacceptable.
- Milk, although it appears to be nutritious and convenient, is usually an expensive source of calories and is perishable and subject to contamination.
- Meal preparation by teachers takes time from teaching and thus from learning.

Some of these problems can be addressed by concentrating supplies on the neediest groups, by offering breakfast and snacks instead of more elaborate meals, by employing outside vendors (including mothers) to supply foods, and by encouraging community participation.

One problem is especially difficult to work around: transporting large quantities of food in countries with poor transportation and communication systems. One option for donated food, called monetization, is to sell the food in the general market so that the central government can give the proceeds to school systems for feeding programs; the school systems then purchase the food in their local communities. Monetization generates income for the local economy, but by putting donated food on the market it can depress indigenous food production, and the process has frequently been a source of mismanagement and corruption.

Enhancing School Feeding Programs

Several actions can boost the educational and nutritional value of school feeding programs:

- Provide the meal or snack early in the school day. The goal is to eliminate hunger so that children are more attentive in class. Children who come to school without breakfast need to eat early in the day to maximize learning.
- Set the caloric quantity and nutritional quality of the ration to meet the actual needs of the children. As a general rule, feeding programs should provide from one-third to one-half of the recommended daily calorie intake of the school-age population, based on the assumption that it replaces one of two or three daily meals. In addition to an adequate number of calories in the ration, it should fill the actual micronutrient gaps in the children's diet.
- Offer other school-based health and nutrition interventions in addition to food. Treating children for parasites, for example, can improve both their appetites and the nutritional benefit of the food ration. If the ration is neither a good source of nutrients nor adequately fortified with them, the feeding program can be used to deliver micronutrient supplements. Nutrition and health education aimed at changing specific nutrition and health practices could also enhance the benefits of school feeding programs (see below on changing children's behavior).

Keeping School Feeding Programs Affordable

To cut the cost of these programs or to initiate them more cheaply, they should be targeted, and community participation should be generated. Targeting programs to schools with the highest proportion of malnourished or hungry children is the key to making programs cost-effective. Among the criteria for identifying the most needy zones or schools can be nutritional status, the results of a height-for-age census, or, if no information is available on malnutrition or hunger, poverty indicators. In any case, programs must minimize the participation of schools that have a large proportion of children who are not hungry or that have the resources to obtain their own food. But once a program chooses a school, experience has shown targeting groups of students *within* it to be impractical and socially unacceptable.

Local communities can participate in school feeding programs and help cut costs by assuming the responsibility for food preparation and delivery. They also can often provide some of the food itself. Raising money through the sale of food grown in school or community gardens may be another route to making school feeding programs more affordable.[4]

Changing School Feeding Programs

Once a program is in place, altering it can meet strong resistance. Among the modifications that might be needed are changing from a midday meal to a breakfast, moving the program from one group of schools to another that is more needy, obtaining more resources from the local community, or shifting meal preparation and delivery to the private sector. Such changes can be opposed both by communities facing the loss of a program or the increased demand for their time to support it and, in the case of privatization, by the governmental department running the program.

Windows of opportunity for change may arise. In the Dominican Republic, a donor-assisted school feeding program has been a reality for more than four decades. But a recent change in the source of support (from the U.S. Agency for International Development to the World Food Programme) was the opportunity to change the program from lunch to breakfast and to transfer it from schools with questionable need to those with high levels of malnutrition (measured by a national height-for-age census). Raising the consciousness of personnel in the education sector about the benefits of change and offering specific advice on what they might do to improve programs helped to overcome resistance.

Promoting Participation by the Private Sector

To reduce the time that feeding programs take away from learning and to ensure a consistent daily ration, many governments have given private enterprises the responsibility for preparing and delivering a ready-to-eat meal or snack. If governments seek large-scale enterprises to take over feeding programs, privatization will displace small food vendors

---

Box 8. Privatized U.S. School Lunches: Better Nutrition at Lower Cost

Converting from a government-supplied to a privately supplied school lunch program in the U.S. state of Rhode Island has led to cheaper yet tastier and more nutritious lunches in the public schools there. The state government recently terminated its twenty-five-year-old program of centrally planned and purchased lunches for the public schools in the state and hired private contractors to take over the program. The annual cost of the program to the state plummeted, from $11 million to $200,000, and federal and state subsidies, combined, fell almost one-half. An expressed concern at the time of the conversion was that a privately run program would emphasize profit over nutritional quality, but the new program delivers higher nutritional value than the old program did, and student participation in the program has soared. (See Glass 1995.)

---

already selling food to students. Instead, governments should encourage small, local enterprises. Some school canteens in Lesotho, for example, are run by former local vendors who successfully bid on the privatized service. In Nigeria state and local governments train and license vendors who sell to schoolchildren. In Indonesia school principals use their considerable power to choose the vendors who serve their schools (Cohen 1991).

Another major concern with privatization is the quality and hygiene of the food served. Governments need to regulate what is sold by commercial vendors and regulate the standards of sanitation. Even in the United States, concern for the nutritional quality of foods provided by private vendors has made the move to privatization slow; yet where it has occurred, the benefits appear to be substantial (see box 8).

The Cost-Effectiveness of School Feeding Programs

Despite decades of experience worldwide and despite the fact that school feeding programs are often criticized for being too expensive, we do not know whether these programs are cost-effective. Surprisingly few high-quality evaluations and analyses have been conducted. A large-scale survey and analysis of ninety-seven programs in Latin America, including school feeding programs, found that only ten had been evaluated, and only three of these had been evaluated adequately (World Bank 1991). Most program information relates to number of children reached rather than to more meaningful measures such as cost per thousand calories transferred over the school year or to the program's effect on nutrition, health, or education.

School feeding programs are a reality in many countries. Without an evaluation of these programs, it is unwise to consider proposals for new programs.

Long-Term Programs

Schools with no supply of clean water and no sanitary facilities are poor locations for health and nutrition programs. And the benefits of health and nutrition programs will be temporary if the opportunity to change children's relevant behavior goes unexploited during their school years.

Improving the School Environment

The school environment may damage the health and nutritional status of schoolchildren if it increases their exposure to hazards such as infectious diseases carried by the water supply. Hygiene education is difficult without clean water. Providing clean water and sanitary facilities may also boost the attendance of girls—the lack of such facilities at school is an important cause of absenteeism during menstruation. Various countries have large-scale programs to improve water supply and sanitation, but these programs may not specifically target schools. Over the long term, water and sanitation and other community and household improvements are critical to sustaining the benefits of short-to-medium-term interventions.

New school construction and the rehabilitation of existing schools should focus on building latrines and systems for access to clean water. School-based promotional and educational efforts could encourage communities to build latrines. Only concrete and reinforcing rods for the slab are required. Improving access to clean water through community-based schemes is more difficult, but promoting the collection of rainwater may be an option in some areas. Teachers and other school personnel involved in school health activities could also help schools link up with donor and governmental resources for developing water and sanitation systems.

Changing Children's Behavior

Inappropriate behavior by school-age children, such as playing in or drinking impure water, is the basis of many of their nutrition and health problems. Education that addresses specific nutrition and health practices is thus a critical element of school health programs. Such education complements, and can help sustain, the benefits of short-to-medium-term interventions such as deworming and micronutrient supplementation.

Although many schools offer education in nutrition and health, the value of these programs usually is uncertain. Promising methods of delivering such education to children, adolescents, and the wider community are the child-to-child (participatory) approach and informational, educational, and communication programs based on the principles of social marketing. Helping children develop life skills—psychosocial or personal skills such as decisionmaking, critical thinking, self-awareness, and problem solving—also has a positive effect on health-related behaviors.

THE CHILD-TO-CHILD APPROACH. Child-to-child, an educational method that originated in Africa, has been tried in almost all African countries as well as in many other countries in the developing world. Child-to-child offers a curriculum for the school-age youngster that (a) does not depend on the didactic relation between teacher and student but rather involves children in health-related activities and (b) sees the children as the conduit for reaching their siblings, parents, and communities. By developing activities for the student outside of school time, child-to-child helps children internalize lessons by putting them into everyday practice and in that way helps spread the lessons beyond the school population.

Despite the abundance of child-to-child programs, few have been evaluated, so their effectiveness is uncertain. Some programs have been credited with raising vaccination rates and others with improving children's hygiene; one long-term evaluation showed significant gains in the children's knowledge of anemia and significant changes in their dietary practices.[5] Innovative programs in Ecuador and Mozambique, for example, offer school activities as part of a promotional campaign accompanying the national iodization of salt. At the schools, children will test salt that they bring from home for iodine content.

SOCIAL MARKETING. Social marketing is the use of commercial marketing techniques for social purposes. In contrast to traditional health education based on the assumption that suboptimal behavior is a function of lack of knowledge, social marketing recognizes and addresses the gap that can divide knowledge and behavior. Consultations with targeted individuals—via, for example, focus group discussions, key informant interviews, classroom and home observations, and household and school trials—provide insights on how people's own values and predilections can be used to motivate them to adopt new behaviors. This process defines not only how to educate people about a specific problem or area but also how to select and implement interventions. The complete strategy also helps to achieve and maintain political support and trains and motivates program implementors and community members (see box 6).

Social marketing has been effective in improving the health and nutrition behaviors of women and also of the caretakers of infants and young children. The approach is just beginning to be applied to parents of school-age children and to the children themselves. In the Dominican Republic and Guinea, for example, ongoing consultations with children, teachers, and parents concern the school and home environment and the behaviors that affect the nutrition and health of school-age children. The goal is the selection and delivery of interventions, supported by a communications and education program, that will alter the practices of the children and their parents.

DEVELOPING CHILDREN'S LIFE SKILLS. Decisionmaking, problem solving, communication, critical thinking, self-assessment, and coping strategies are called life skills. When people have such skills, they are more likely to adopt a healthy lifestyle. Older school-age children with such skills have been shown to resist such risk-taking behaviors as precocious or unsafe sex.

Schools can help young people acquire life skills. In Mexico, for example, adolescent boys who took part in a life skills sex education program before they became sexually active were much more likely to use contraceptives in later relationships than those who had not taken part. In the United States, a skills-based health education curriculum was shown to significantly increase health knowledge among elementary school students and, among secondary school students, to achieve reductions in self-reported drug use, alcohol consumption, and cigarette smoking (Connell, Turner, and Mason 1985). Although no research has been conducted on life skills education in Africa, the HIV/AIDS pandemic has led Uganda and Zimbabwe to put life skills training into their school programs.

Notes

1. The kit would contain disinfectant for wounds, an analgesic, packets of oral rehydration solution (ORS) for diarrhea, treatment for scabies, and possibly antimalarial drugs.

2. A WHO/UNICEF program, Integrated Management of the Sick Child, has developed a protocol for the detection of fever by touch if no thermometer is available and for the detection of clinical signs indicating the need for antimalarial drugs. The protocol would be useful in the schools.

3. It may be possible to alleviate hunger in schoolchildren without a formal feeding program. Encouraging and educating parents to feed their children before

sending them to school or to provide money for them to purchase food while at school may be one alternative.

4. Gardens are not usually intended to provide food directly to programs, and many constraints must be overcome or bypassed if gardens are to be successful. In particular, gardening must not be allowed to unduly burden students or take away from their instruction time.

5. Children interviewed five years after they completed a school-based child-to-child program on anemia, diarrhea, and immunization were more knowledgeable about the clinical features of anemia (66 percent compared with 0 percent of children who had not participated in the program), about its treatment (42 percent compared with 0 percent), and about its prevention (80 percent compared with 2 percent). The consumption of appropriate iron-containing foods also was more regular among children who participated in the program—56 percent compared with 24 percent, based on self-reported consumption (Lansdowne 1995).

5

The Lessons Learned

The steady rise in demand and support for school nutrition and health programs over the past few years has generated many new efforts. Experience with these efforts to date does not provide any firm conclusions about best practice. Nonetheless, lessons have been learned that can guide those charged with developing school nutrition and health programs.

Coordinating Resources

With the burgeoning attention and resources devoted to school health and nutrition programs comes the need to coordinate efforts that otherwise could be redundant, wasteful, or—worse—unsuccessful. The good news is that, with the many sources of support available today, the opportunities are there to complement donor programs with a combination of features previously unavailable.

Parallel developments in United Nations Children's Fund (UNICEF) and World Bank programs illustrate the opportunities for coordination. Over the past several years UNICEF has dedicated considerable attention to adolescent health and development in Burundi, Cameroon, Sri Lanka, Thailand, and Zimbabwe, with a focus on teenage pregnancy, smoking and substance abuse, violence, and the prevention and control of sexually transmitted diseases. More recently, UNICEF has broadened its school health focus to a school-based health package that also addresses problems of younger school-age children (see box 9).

At the same time, support at the World Bank for school-based nutrition and health efforts has grown substantially. During fiscal 1983–88 virtually no World Bank education project included nutrition and health, whereas such concerns were a feature of almost half the education projects approved during fiscal 1988–96 (see appendix B). These activities range from the construction of school canteens to school health programs that include examinations, feeding, micronutrient supplementation, and deworming. In some countries UNICEF and other donors are better organized and equipped than the World Bank to provide on-the-ground supervision of and support for implementation of these programs. School health and nutrition initiatives in Burkina

---

Box 9. UNICEF's School Health Program

Health and Nutrition Services

- Screening for common health problems
- Prevention and treatment of common health problems; first aid
- Linkages and referral between schools and health services
- School feeding programs

Knowledge and Skills for Health

- Curriculum development for skills-based education
- Extracurricular school health activities, such as school health clubs or child-to-child activities
- Physical education and sports

A Healthy and Supportive Environment

- Clean water and sanitation in schools
- Policies for ethical relations between teachers and students; for example, support for pregnant girls
- Positive psychosocial environment

Faso are just such an instance in which the World Bank and UNICEF have advantageously combined efforts (see box 10). Not only is UNICEF providing complementary program elements, it is also helping to work out the difficulties posed by a lack of coordination within the national government (see the following section).

Other donors are also investing more in school nutrition and health programs. The Health Education and Promotion Division of the World Health Organization (WHO), which serves as the coordinating point for twenty-two WHO divisions, supports many school-based health education activities. WHO recently convened a meeting of experts on school-age children's health to introduce its new school-based health initiative, which supports health services, improvements in the school environment, and health education. The World Food Programme offers another kind of resource: substantial amounts of donated food for school feeding programs. Coordinating these resources will maximize their effect. The United Nations Educational, Scientific, and Cultural Organization (UNESCO) has emphasized the impact of environmental and food problems on the school-aged and on their school participation rates. In selected countries, UNESCO has assessed the healthfulness of the school environment, has monitored children's nutritional status and school progress, and has assessed such learning and working conditions in schools as class size, lighting, noise, furniture, and learning materials. In addition, the Rockefeller Foundation, the Edna McConnell Clark Foundation, and the James S. McDonnell Foundation all support the Partnership for Child Development. The Partnership currrently mobilizes resources for school health and nutrition programs and supports such programs in six countries (Colombia, Ghana, India, Indonesia, Tanzania, and Vietnam).

Linking the Health and Education Sectors

The health and education sectors must ultimately work together in providing nutrition and health programs to school-age children. Although school feeding programs are usually delivered exclusively through one sector or the other, the most efficient and effective means of delivering the broadest range of services is through collaboration between these sectors. Lack of such collaboration has been a major stumbling block in implementing school nutrition and health programs. In Mozambique, for example, a health component of an education project assisted by the World Bank has completely stalled because of the failure of the ministries of health and education to work together. The same problem plagues the health component of the Burkina Faso project (see preceding section and box 10). As an interim measure, UNICEF is stepping in to provide the necessary coordination in both countries. Coordination need not always be so difficult. In Guinea, for example, the school health department is housed in the Ministry of Education but is staffed by health personnel who report to the Ministry of Health. Bolivia has created a supraministry, the Ministry of Human Development, to facilitate intersectoral programming. These arrangements can ease collaboration.

Collaboration can take many forms depending on the strengths of individual ministries. Ghana, assisted by the Partnership for Child

---

Box 10. World Bank–UNICEF Collaboration in Burkino Faso

The government of Burkina Faso and UNICEF have signed an agreement to improve the nutrition and health of school-age children, with World Bank assistance. The Bank, which drew attention to the critical nutritional and health needs of the children, gave technical assistance to Burkina Faso's subsequent plan to address those needs as part of the country's program to improve primary education as a whole. UNICEF will provide much-needed on-the-ground support for the nutrition and health component by identifying a local coordinator, aiding the collaboration between the ministries of health and education, and assisting with drug procurement, the development of health education programs, and monitoring and evaluation.

Development, is implementing a program of anthelmintic treatment and health education through the Ministry of Education with technical assistance provided by the Ministry of Health. Taking advantage of the health sector infrastructure, the drug distribution system delivers tablets to the central medical stores or to the parasitic diseases unit of the Ministry of Health and from there to regional medical stores. They are then repackaged, sent to the district education office, and finally distributed to schools by circuit officers of the educational sector. Teachers are trained by health sector personnel to administer drugs, and they also receive pamphlets describing what to do.

Taking a different tack toward coordination, Tanzania's Ministry of Health is operating an anthelmintic program through its National School Health program, which in turn has coordinators from both the health and education ministries at all levels. Drugs are to be delivered through a chain of medical stores, where they are repackaged and ultimately delivered to the schools. Health personnel will train teachers to administer the drugs.

A Feasible Package of Services

The concept that schools can deliver a package of health services to students is now widely acknowledged. The appropriate level of services for schools to offer in any given country will be a function of what is operationally and financially feasible. The World Bank's *World Development Report* on health identifies a limited package of cost-effective school-based health services: control of parasitic worms, micronutrient interventions, and health education (World Bank 1993). The broader public health package recommended in the report also covers other issues—family planning and nutrition, tobacco and alcohol consumption, the environment, HIV/AIDS—in which schools have a potential role to play through social marketing programs and education-for-life skills.

UNICEF has recommended a more comprehensive and detailed package of school-based health and nutrition services, but it acknowledges that the particular set of interventions or services offered in any given country will depend on what is feasible and affordable. Some countries will be capable of developing a broad range of services. In the state of São Paulo, Brazil, which has a relatively long history of providing nutrition and health programs through the schools, a World Bank loan is helping to improve school feeding programs, to implement health and nutrition screening of schoolchildren, to integrate nutrition and health education into the school curriculum, and to implement school-based programs for iron and vitamin A supplementation. Similarly, the government of the Dominican Republic, which also has many years of experience with school feeding programs and a well-developed infrastructure, has received World Bank support for the distribution of iron-fortified snacks in poor urban areas, a national height census of first graders, a national survey of micronutrient deficiencies, the integration of education with feeding, and the development of school-based deworming programs.

Other situations call for a more limited package of services, focusing on interventions that are low-cost and easy to implement. Guinea has had almost no nutrition and health programming for school-age children. Its communication and transportation systems are not well developed, and the local capacity for implementing school-based nutrition and health services is extremely weak. In such a situation, the most critical nutrition and health needs of school-age children have priority. Through a World Bank loan, the elements of a national school-based health package that are to be implemented first are a deworming program and an iron and iodine supplementation program, accompanied by education in health and hygiene. Additional elements—such as malaria treatment and first aid through schools—will be tried on a small scale and added as capacity for their management increases.

Building Local Capacity and Support

Local expertise is indispensable to effective programs; but because school-based health and nutrition programming has been neglected for so long, this expertise is rarely available. The attention and resources now devoted to school-based nutrition and health services will help develop local expertise. Local personnel will benefit, for example, from the experience of developing and implementing situation analyses and relevant interventions; local training is an important element of these activities. Staff participation in international workshops, and other opportunities for sharing experience across countries, will also strengthen local capacity.

Communities and schools play a major role in identifying and solving problems. Africa has a major advantage in the wealth of its community associations; parent-teacher associations, for example, far outnumber health centers. These associations, bolstered by technical support, are the channel for community participation and responsibility. Early involvement in developing a program will maximize the community's commitment to it, which in turn is a key to the program's sustainability. Such early involvement should not be hard to come by: experience shows that local communities want nutrition and health services for school-age children. Communities in Guinea, for example, revealed not only their interest in alleviating the health and nutrition problems of their school-age children but also a willingness to help pay for these services.

Today's Evaluation, Tomorrow's Success

Much remains to be learned. Only by monitoring and evaluating school nutrition and health programs can knowledge grow about what works, at what cost, and under what circumstances. Evaluations of programs need to consider both their health and nutrition effects and their effects on education indicators such as enrollment, attendance, and achievement. Through such monitoring and evaluation, donors and governments will be able to adapt programs to almost any situation, discovering the most cost-effective and feasible approaches to meet the nutrition and health needs of school-age children.

Appendix A
Information Required for a Situation
Analysis of the Nutrition and Health
of School-Age Children

The goal of this situation analysis is to guide the design and evaluation of school-based health and nutrition programs. A situation analysis can be detailed and comprehensive, but the most appropriate initial approach is usually a low-cost, rapid survey that supplies the preliminary answers necessary for intelligent efforts to develop or strengthen school nutrition and health programs.

In the approach outlined here, the situation analysis gathers information sufficient for a report that:

- Identifies the priority nutrition and health problems of school-age children
- Quantifies school participation (enrollment, absenteeism, repetition, and dropout rates) and identifies the major causes of nonattendance
- Identifies the practicable, sustainable interventions that are likely to most improve children's nutrition, health, school attendance, and learning capacity
- Identifies both the major problems with existing school nutrition and health services and the gaps in those services and suggests remedies
- Informs efforts to monitor and evaluate school nutrition and health services
- Identifies issues requiring further investigation.

Information gathering and report writing, in addition, provide an opportunity to establish forward-looking partnerships among school and health personnel and school-age children and youth. Such relationships are an immense help to programs furthering school nutrition and health services. The information for the analysis comes from an assessment of existing information, interviews with key informants, focus group discussions, and other assessment techniques. Information gathering is discussed below under separate headings relating to distinct issues; in practice, however, each assessment, interview, or discussion pursues these issues simultaneously.

Further technical assessment will be required before any new program can arise from the initial assessment report. In particular, more refined targeting of interventions will undoubtedly require more specific analyses, including biomedical surveys. Given the context of advocacy in which any situation analysis is written, it should present its information in an interesting and accessible manner and use a variety of data to give depth and emphasis. For example, a comparison of the share of household income spent on smoking and alcohol with the share spent on the health care of school-age children might add force to the portrait drawn by the report.

Identifying Priority Nutrition and Health Problems

The Information Required

Causes of morbidity and mortality. Information on the major causes of death and illness is fundamental to the selection of priority interventions. The data must also include health problems that begin in childhood and adolescence but that manifest themselves only later in life—HIV infection, for example. Besides the causes of disease and death, the information should ideally include the age and sex of victims, the urbanization and geographic region of their location, and the season during which they were stricken so that interventions designed subsequent to the situation analysis can be carefully targeted. In reality, however, many of these details will not be available.

Trends in mortality and morbidity. Identifying whether a problem is increasing or decreasing through time aids the identification of future priorities.

The extent of short-term hunger and malnutrition. The analysis must pay special attention to nutrition problems and hunger that may not show up in health data and information.

Changes in patterns of health-related behaviors. The analysis should determine whether risky behaviors such as smoking, substance abuse, and precocious or unsafe sex are leading to increases in incidents of violence and unwanted pregnancies.

Other impairments inhibiting school performance. The analysis should gather information on the prevalence of sensory deficits (hearing or vision impairments) and other handicaps among school-age children.

The role of social and cultural factors as health determinants. The relationship of identified nutrition and health problems to current societal values and norms is important for the design of programs, especially in regard to the health of girls.

Locating the Information Required

Reports and surveys in the international and national literature. Technical support groups might review the international literature; local research institutes, the national literature. Sources of information beyond the education and health sectors can be useful. For example, the criminal justice area may provide information relevant to adolescent behavior patterns. Information is particularly required for patterns of:

- Mortality by cause
- Micronutrient deficiency (vitamin A, iron, iodine)
- Anthropometrics (height-for-age and weight-for-height measures) and other measures of nutritional status
- Short-term hunger
- Parasitic infections, including malaria and worm infection
- Early pregnancy, reproductive health (sexually transmitted diseases, HIV/AIDS, reproductive tract infections, menstrual health), and tetanus in adolescents
- Sexual exploitation and abuse
- Respiratory infections, including tuberculosis
- Recurrent or intermittent fevers, including those from malaria and acute respiratory infection (ARI)
- Immunizable diseases (polio, tetanus, typhoid)
- Hearing and sight impairment
- Skin infections
- Dental problems
- Chronic disability and mental illness
- Violence, accidents, and dependency on alcohol, tobacco, and drugs.

Routine mortality and morbidity statistics. Data on the causes of admission and outpatient attendance at hospitals, clinics, and other local medical centers are inevitably biased by the catchment area and user group, but they provide information on utilization. Data from casualty centers may be the only source of information on violence and accidents.

Interviews. Informants include staff members of the ministries of health and education and of nongovernmental organizations (NGOs) focused on health or youths, relevant university faculty, health professionals, and officials in the criminal justice system. The interviews, perhaps based on the above list of conditions, would seek to rank the causes of ill health according to national patterns and major variations.

Questionnaires and focus group discussions. These can determine the perceptions of teachers, health workers, parents, and students about major nutrition and health problems. Such questionnaires and discussions may clarify whether the community perception of the causation and distribution of nutrition and health problems differs from empirical observation. As with information on the intersection of social norms and health-related behaviors, knowledge of perceptions is essential to the development of appropriate nutrition and health education messages. The discussions also permit an assessment of psychosocial factors, such as stress, particularly in the broader social context described by the standard UNICEF situation analysis (for example, unemployment and social disruption). The questionnaires and focus groups may also provide background information on patterns of sexual abuse, which would usefully be supplemented indirectly by age-specific measures of sexually transmitted diseases.

Using Schools to Reach the School-Age Group

The Information Required

The size of the school-age population, enrollment and dropout rates, and the proportion of children repeating grades. This information identifies predominant patterns in education sector indicators. The data should cover the primary and secondary levels and variations by age or grade, sex, urbanization, and region.

Absenteeism rates. The analysis must gather information—by age, sex, urbanization, and region, as well as by season and day of the week—on the proportion of children who are formally enrolled in school and regularly fail to attend. In some regions the seasons of high agricultural activity have high rates of absenteeism and would be particularly inappropriate times for school-based delivery of interventions. Likewise, extensive absenteeism on a regular market day would be revealed by statistics on absenteeism by day of the week.

Causes of nonenrollment and absenteeism. The primary causes of absenteeism may not be among the major health issues, but identifying ways to reduce absenteeism is critical if children are to receive schooling and school-based nutrition and health interventions.

The potential role of nonformal education. Information on the extent of the nonformal education sector may reveal further opportunities to deliver nutrition and health education and services. The nonformal sector may be important for particular groups, such as girls or adolescents, that may be underserved by the formal sector.

Laws and policies relevant to school-age children. Information should cover laws on sexual harassment by teachers, laws on limiting youths' access to tobacco and alcohol, policies on sex education, and policies on allowing school-age girls who become pregnant to return to school.

Current community spending on the education, nutrition, and health of school-age children. This information will indicate the potential for school nutrition and health programs to achieve sustainability through community contributions and other community approaches to cost recovery.

Locating the Information Required

Reports and surveys in the international and national literature. The national literature, particularly from the ministry of education, is likely to be the most valuable.

Statistics assembled by regional and district education services. Most of the assembled data are collated from summaries sent in from local levels. Thus the detailed data are held at the local levels, but their analysis may require special expertise such as that in local education research institutions.

Interviews. See the section above on nutrition and health.

Summaries of collected data. Summaries can be shared with teachers, other workers in the health and education sectors, and older students, who can say whether the data identify the important determinants of enrollment and absenteeism. These discussions will further help identify the determinants. Special efforts will be required to interview youths who are not enrolled, or who are frequently absent, and their parents, but such interviews would be especially likely to reveal current practices and perceptions relating to laws and policies.

Assessing the Capacity to Promote and Implement Programs

The Information Required

Existing nutrition and health services for school-age children. Of interest are not only existing school programs but also general health services that school-age children are intended to use. Information on the availability of material and financial resources will be particularly important in assessing local resource capacity and response. Basic topics include:

- The relative responsibilities of the health and education sectors for school nutrition and health education and services
- National and regional policies bearing on school nutrition and health programs—their relevance and the extent to which they are open for review
- The structure, components, and coverage of any existing school nutrition and health programs, including the customary health screening and first aid programs
- Current approaches to health education, including family life and reproductive health education and other nutrition- and health-related activities, such as school health clubs
- Current use of primary health care facilities by the school-age group, including use of reproductive health facilities and referrals between schools and the primary health care system
- The extent to which school-age children use private health services and traditional healers
- The content, coverage, effectiveness, and cost of school feeding programs and school gardens
- Information on school canteens and local food vendors who serve schools
- Information on school water supply and sanitary and waste disposal facilities
- The contribution of NGOs and intergovernmental organizations to school programs
- The community's contribution to schools and to the provision of clean water and good sanitation facilities, school feeding, and other nutrition and health services
- Current levels of investment by government or other agencies in the health and nutrition of school-age children
- Preschool and special education programming.

Plans for extending services for school-age children. It is necessary to project the availability of resources and the technical and institutional capacity for these purposes.

- Interviews of key individuals and institutions with relevant expertise and interest
- Assessments of the relative strengths and weaknesses of lead agencies and other participating organizations in school health and nutrition programs.

The capacity of the education sector to help deliver nutrition and health education and services. An emphasis on cost data will help in the assessment of program affordability and sustainability. Required information includes:

- The number and distribution of primary and secondary schools and teachers, including a comparison with the number of clinics and health workers
- The content of existing nutrition and health education in schools, including focus, methods, materials, and an overview of relevant curriculums currently being explored or implemented
- The capacity of teacher training institutions to provide training in nutrition and health, including the frequency and coverage of in-service training for teachers
- The contribution of religious organizations and other NGOs to the education sector and their capacity to help deliver nutrition and health education and services
- The contribution of intergovernmental organizations to school nutrition and health programs
- The willingness and capacity of government, other agencies in the education sector, and communities to invest in the nutrition and health of the school-age population
- The willingness and capacity of teachers and schools to play an active role in delivering nutrition and health education and services
- The capacity of the school environment to support health promotion, including the availability at school of clean water and of facilities for menstruating girls.

The existing UNICEF situation analyses of the education and health sectors could contain information on some of these items or could provide a basis for comparison. For example, one informative comparison would be that between the quality of water and sanitation in the school and the quality of water and sanitation within the household and the community.

Current availability of resources. These resources will come from the many sectors relevant to health and education (governmental, nongovernmental, and intergovernmental) and even from the children themselves and from the wider community. Information is also necessary on the financial and economic cost of proposed interventions.

Availability of resources from other entities. These entities include sports and religious organizations, social welfare groups, and the news media. Contributions from such sources may be particularly important in ensuring sustainability.

Locating the Information Required

Reports from the local health and education sectors. These may include quantitative and qualitative information on the number and distribution of schools, clinics, and personnel (including mapping).

Data on resource availability at all stages of analysis described above (report analysis, key informant interviews, discussion groups). Evaluating the cost-effectiveness of specific interventions may require additional studies once a package of interventions has been identified.

Interviews. Interviews with key informants are likely to be the main source of information in this area.

Meetings with representative groups of teachers, teachers' organizations, and other education personnel. These meetings can be used to assess the willingness of education personnel to participate in school nutrition and health programs and to obtain their assessment of the ability of the education sector to accommodate such programs in the face of competing demands for limited resources.

Understanding Perceptions of Program Participants

The Information Required

The community's perspective on school nutrition and health programs. Information on the perceptions of students, parents, teachers, health workers, and others who need to be directly involved in a school nutrition or health program includes perceptions about what needs to be done and about the acceptability and capability of the school system as a source of health and nutrition education and services.

The community's willingness and capacity to support school nutrition and health programs. The issues here are whether students and parents would be willing and able to contribute resources to the development of services and what the scale and type of this contribution would be.

The potential for children to be active participants in improving their nutrition, health, and education. This assessment requires an understanding of existing knowledge, attitudes, beliefs, and practices about health and education.

Locating the Information Required

Discussions with community groups, especially parents' associations, to identify community perceptions.

Interviews.

Note

This protocol was developed by the Partnership for Child Development, a joint initiative of the Rockefeller Foundation and the United Nations Development Programme. The Partnership is now also supported by the Edna McConnell Clark Foundation, the James S. McDonnell Foundation, the Wellcome Trust, the British Overseas Development Administration, the International Development Research Centre, the World Bank, and the United Nations Children's Fund. The Partnership was established in 1992 to improve the health and education of school-age children. The Scientific Coordinating Center for the Partnership is housed in the Center for the Epidemiology of Infectious Disease at Oxford University.

Appendix B
World Bank Projects with Services Related to the Nutrition and Health of School-Age Children, by Country

Country and project	Project period	Service	Cost ($M)
Angola, First Education	1992–2000	Health and nutrition education in curriculum	a
Bangladesh, General Education	1990–98	School feeding (implementation support); nutrition education in curriculum; nonformal nutrition education for parents	a
Bangladesh, Secondary School Assistance	1994–2001	Hygiene education; water and sanitation for schools	1.3
Bolivia, Social Investment Fund	1990–98	School meals (targeted at ages 3–12)	b
Brazil, Innovations in Basic Education	1992–99	School meals (management and training); health screening (vision and hearing); immunizations; preventive oral health; iron and vitamin A supplements; evaluation of nutrition and health interventions	53
Brazil, Northeast Basic Education	1993–2000	Evaluation of school lunch program	0.5
Burkina Faso, Education	1992–2000	Nutrition and health education in curriculum; iodine and vitamin A supplements; deworming; wells and sanitary facilities for schools; impact evaluation of nutrition and health programs	0.5

(Table continues on the following page.)

Appendix B *(continued)*

Country and project	Project period	Service	Cost ($M)
Cape Verde, Education and Training	1995–2002	Operational research on school feeding and other school-based health and nutrition interventions	0.13
Chad, Education Rehabilitation	1990–98	Research on impact of school-based health services; impact evaluation of school canteens	c
Chile, Primary Education Improvement	1993–2001	Health and nutrition screening and referral; school health manual and teacher training; school feeding for preschoolers	5.7
Costa Rica, Basic Education Rehabilitation	1992–2000	Health education in curriculum; teacher training in health education	a
Dominican Republic, Basic Education I	1991–96	Institutional capacity building in nutrition and health services; expansion and targeting of school meals; deworming; social marketing–based health and nutrition education; iron-fortified school breakfasts	1.6
Dominican Republic, Basic Education II	1996–2002	School nutrition and health services as under Basic Education I (school feeding, deworming, micronutrients, and capacity building)	3.2
Ecuador, Social Development	1992–98	Research on nutrition, health, and education	c
El Salvador, Structural Adjustment I	1991–98	Fortified school biscuits for primary schools	b
El Salvador, Basic Education Modernization	1996–2002	Deworming; vitamin A and iodine supplementation; health screening and referral through schools; social marketing–based health education	1.5
Equatorial Guinea, Primary Education	1988–94	School canteen construction	a
Guatemala, Basic Education	1989–96	Food storerooms and kitchen construction	a

Country and project	Project period	Service	Cost ($M)
Guinea, Equity and School Improvement	1996–2002	Deworming; iodine supplementation; pilot-level iron supplementation and malaria treatment; social marketing–based health education; situation analyses of school nutrition and health; capacity building in school nutrition and health	1.8
Honduras, Social Investment Fund	1991–96	School breakfast, targeted through parent-teacher associations (PTAs)	b
Lesotho, Education Sector Development	1992–98	Impact evaluation of school gardens	c
Madagascar, Education Reinforcement	1990–97	Nutrition education in curriculum	a
Mali, Education Consolidation	1989–96	Nutrition education in primary curriculum	a
Morocco, Rural Primary Education	1989–96	School health services (technical equipment); health and nutrition education in curriculum; teacher training in health education; advanced training in school health	1.7
Morocco, Rural Basic Education	1991–98	School canteen construction; school meals (subsidized); evaluation of school feeding	a
Mozambique, Education II	1991–98	School rehabilitation; latrine construction; pilot-level deworming and iron supplementation; school feeding (expansion); institutional development for school health	0.2
Niger, Basic Education	1995–2001	School-based deworming; micronutrient supplementation via schools; health and hygiene education; institutional development for school health	0.4

(Table continues on the following page.)

Appendix B *(continued)*

Country and project	Project period	Service	Cost ($M)
Pakistan, Sind Primary Education	1990–98	School feeding (local foods, via PTAS); evaluation of school feeding	3.5
Peru, Health and Nutrition	1994–2000	Deworming	0.3
Philippines, Elementary Education	1991–99	School breakfasts (improvements through education and community involvement)	0.3
Poland, Structural Adjustment	1991–96	Evaluation of school feeding	c
Solomon Islands, Education and Training III	1994–2001	Training for school nurses	1.0
Sri Lanka, Economic Restructuring	1991–98	Midday meal (restructuring; food stamps through schools)	b
Venezuela, Structural Adjustment	1989–95	Consolidation of school feeding programs	b
Zaire, Education Rehabilitation	1990–97	Teacher training in health, nutrition, and hygiene; nonformal nutrition education for parents	a
Zambia, Education Rehabilitation	1993–2000	Health and hygiene education; study on cholera and environmental health in schools	a

a. Fully integrated with curriculum development efforts or construction activities under the project; separate cost cannot be determined.

b. Cost of specific elements of structural adjustment and social investment funds operations cannot be disaggregated to this level.

c. Less than 0.1 million.

References

Bautista, Arturo, P. A. Barker, J. T. Dunn, M. Sanchez, and D. L. Kaiser. 1982. "The Effects of Iodized Oil on Intelligence, Thyroid Status, and Somatic Growth in School-Age Children from an Area of Endemic Goiter." *American Journal of Clinical Nutrition* 35: 127–34.

Bleichrodt, N., P. J. D. Drenth, and A. Querido. 1980. "Effects of Iodine Deficiency on Mental and Psychomotor Abilities." *American Journal of Physical Anthropology* 53: 55–67.

Bleichrodt, N., I. Garcia, C. Rubio, G. Morreale de Escobar, and F. Escobar del Rey. 1987. "Developmental Disorders Associated with Severe Iodine Deficiency." In B. S. Hetzel, J. T. Dunn, and J. B. Stanbury, eds., *The Prevention and Control of IDD*. New York: Elsevier.

Bloem, M. W., M. Wedel, E. J. van Agtmaal, A. J. Speck, S. Saowakortha, and W. H. P. Schreurs. 1990. "Vitamin A Intervention: Short-Term Effects of a Single Massive Dose on Iron Metabolism." *American Journal of Clinical Nutrition* 51: 76–79.

Brabin, Loretta, and Bernard J. Brabin. 1992. "The Cost of Successful Adolescent Growth and Development in Girls in Relation to Iron and Vitamin A Status." *American Society for Clinical Nutrition* 55: 995–98.

Bundy, D. A. P., M. S. Wong, L. L. Lewis, and J. Horton. 1990. "Control of Helminths by Delivery of Targeted Chemotherapy through Schools." *Transactions of the Royal Society of Tropical Medicine and Hygiene* 84: 115–20.

Butler, James C., and Philip J. Porter. 1994. "School-Based Health Services for Children and Families in the USA: Experience from 1965 to 1994." World Bank, Human Development Department, Washington, D.C.

Catholic Relief Services. 1993a. "Ghana Program: Multi-Year Operational Plan, 1994–96." Baltimore, Md.

———. 1993b. "Ghana Program, Title II PL480, Progress Report." Baltimore, Md.

Ceci, Stephen. 1995. Unpublished data. Cornell University, Department of Nutrition, Ithaca, N.Y.

Chwang, L. C., A. G. Soemantri, and Ernesto Pollitt. 1988. "Iron Supplementation and Physical Growth of Rural Indonesian Children." *American Journal of Clinical Nutrition* 47: 496–501.

Cohen, Monique. 1991. "Use of Microenterprises in the Delivery of Food Programs to School Children." World Bank, Population and Human Resources Department, Washington, D.C.

Connell, David F., Ralph R. Turner, and Elaine F. Mason. 1985. "Summary of Findings of the School Health Education Evaluation: Health Promotion Effectiveness, Implementation, and Costs." *Journal of School Health* 55: 316–21.

Devadas, R. P. 1983. *The Honorable Chief Minister's Nutritious Meal Programme for Children of Tamil Nadu*. Coimbatore, India: Sri Arinashilingam Home Science College.

Florencio, C. A. 1987. "Impact of Nutrition on the Academic Achievement and Other School-Related Behaviors of Grade One through Six Pupils." University of the Philippines, Manila.

Glass, Stephen. 1995. "Incredible Yet Edible: How Rhode Island Beefed Up Its School Lunch Program." *Washington Post* (September 3).

Glewwe, Paul, and Hanan Jacoby. 1994. *An Economic Analysis of Delayed Primary School Enrollment and Childhood Nutrition in Ghana.* LSMS Working Paper 98. World Bank, Washington, D.C.

Gopaldas, Tara, and Sunder Gujral. 1996. "The Pre-Post Impact Evaluation of the Improved Mid-Day-Meal Programme, Gujarat." Tara Consultancy Services, Baroda, India.

Grantham-McGregor, Sally. 1993. "Assessments of the Effects of Nutrition on Mental Development and Behavior in Jamaican Studies." *American Journal of Clinical Nutrition* 57 (suppl.): 303S–9S.

Griffiths, Marcia, and Mike Favin. 1993. "Social Marketing of Insecticide-Treated Bed Nets for Malaria Control Programs." Manoff Group, Washington, D.C.

Gupta, M. C., and K. Hom. 1984. "Evaluation of PL480 Title II School Feeding Program in India: Evaluation Report 1984." United States Agency for International Development, Washington, D.C.

Harbison, Ralph W., and Eric A. Hanushek. 1992. *Educational Performance of the Poor: Lessons from Rural Northeast Brazil.* New York: Oxford University Press.

Horton, Susan. 1992. "Unit Costs, Cost-Effectiveness, and Financing of Nutrition Interventions." PHN Working Paper 952. World Bank, Human Development Department, Washington, D.C.

Houde-Nadeau, Michèle, and D. Hunter. N.d. "Nutrition and School Performance in Canadian Children from Low Socio-Economic Areas." University of Montreal, Quebec.

Israel, Ronald, Margaret Wilson, and Alexandra Praun. N.d. "Lessons Learned: The First Country Analysis of the Nutrition, Health, and Related Learning Needs of Primary School Students in Developing Countries." Education Development Center, Action Group for International School Nutrition and Health, Newton, Mass.

Jacoby, Enrique, Santiago Cueto, and Ernesto Pollitt. N.d. "Evaluation of a School Breakfast Program among Andean Children in Huaraz Peru." Instituto de Investigacion Nutricional, Lima, Peru.

Jamison, Dean. 1985. "Child Malnutrition and School Performance in China." EDT 17. World Bank, Education and Training Department, Washington, D.C.

Jamison, Dean T., and W. Henry Mosley, with Anthony R. Measham and José Luis Bobadilla, eds. 1993. *Disease Control Priorities in Developing Countries.* New York: Oxford University Press.

Jarousse, Jean Pierre, and Alain Mingat. 1991. "Assistance a la formulation d'une politique nationale et d' un programme d'investissement dans le secteur de l'education au Benin." Projet UNESCO/PNUD Benin/89/001. Paris: United Nations Educational, Scientific, and Cultural Organization.

King, Joyce. 1990. "Evaluation of School Feeding in the Dominican Republic." CARE, Santo Domingo, Dominican Republic.

Kotchabhakdi, N., P. Hathirat, A. Valyasevi, and E. Pollitt. 1989. "Biological and Social Factors Related to School Performance in Thai Children." Mahidol University, Bangkok, Thailand; University of California, Davis.

Lansdowne, Richard. 1995. "Child-to-Child: A Review of the Literature." Child-to-Child Trust Institute of Education, London.

McDonald, M. A., Mariam Sigman, Michael P. Espinosa, and Charlotte G. Neumann. 1994. "Impact of Temporary Food Shortage on Children and Their Mothers." *Child Development* 65: 404–15.

Meyers, Alan, Amy Sampson, and Michael Weitzman. 1989. "School Breakfast Program and School Performance." *American Journal of Development of Children* 143: 1234–39.

Moock, Peter R., and Joanne Leslie. 1986. "Childhood Malnutrition and Schooling in the Terai Region of Nepal." *Journal of Development Economics* 20: 33–52.

Moore, Emily. 1994. "Evaluation of the Burkina Faso School Feeding Program." Catholic Relief Services, Baltimore, Md.

Murray, C. J. L., and A. D. Lopez. 1994. *Global Comparative Assessments in the Health Sector: Disease Burden, Expenditures, and Intervention Packages.* Geneva: World Health Organization.

Nokes, C., S. M. Grantham-McGregor, A. W. Sawyer, E. S. Cooper, and D. A. P. Bundy. 1992a. "Helminth Infection and Cognitive Function." *Proceedings of the Royal Society* (London) 247: 77–81.

Nokes, Catharine, S. M. Grantham-McGregor, A. W. Sawyer, E. S. Cooper, B. A. Robinson, and D. A. P. Bundy. 1992b. "Moderate to Heavy Infections of *Trichuris trichiura* Affect Cognitive Function in Jamaican School Children." *Parasitology* 104: 539–47.

Pollitt, Ernesto, K. Gorman, E. Engle, R. Martorell, and J. Rivera. 1993. *Early Supplementary Feeding and Cognition: Effects over Two Decades.* Society for Research in Child Development Monograph 235. Chicago: University of Chicago Press.

Rothman, Margaret, and Janet Collins. Forthcoming. "The Potential Costs and Benefits of Selected Components of a Comprehensive School Health Education Program." Centers for Disease Control, Department of Health Education, Atlanta, Ga. Submitted to the *Journal of School Health.*

Seshadri, S., and T. Gopaldas. 1989. "Impact of Iron Supplementation on Cognitive Functions in Pre-School and School-Aged Children: The Indian Experience." *American Journal of Clinical Nutrition* 50 (suppl.): 675–84.

Shrestha, Ramesh Man. 1994. "Effects of Iodine and Iron Supplementation on Physical, Psychomotor, and Mental Development in Primary School Children in Malawi." Ph.D. thesis, University of Malawi, Wapeningen.

Sigman, Mariam, Charlotte Neumann, Ake A. J. Jansen, and Nimrod Bwibo. 1989. "Cognitive Abilities of Kenyan Children in Relation to Nutrition, Family Characteristics, and Education." *Child Development* 60: 1463–74.

Simeon, D. T., and S. Grantham-McGregor. 1989. "Effects of Missing Breakfast on Cognitive Function of Schoolchildren of Differing Nutritional Status." *American Journal of Clinical Nutrition* 49: 646–53.

Stephenson, Lani, Michael Latham, Elizabeth J. Adams, Stephen N. Kinoti, and Anne Peutet. 1989. "Treatment with a Single Dose of Albendazole Improves Growth of Kenyan School Children with Hookworm, *Trichuris Trichiura,* and *Ascaris Lumbricoides* Infection." *American Journal of Tropical Medicine and Hygiene* 41: 78–87.

Tagwireyi, Julia, and Ted Greiner. 1994. *Nutrition in Zimbabwe: An Update.* Washington, D.C.: World Bank.

UNESCO (United Nations Educational, Scientific, and Cultural Organization). N.d.
    Food Aid for Education: UNESCOs Cooperation with the World Food Program. Paris.
UNICEF (United Nations Children's Fund). 1995. "Price List, Jan.–June 1995."
    Essential Drugs, Supply Division, UNICEF, Copenhagen.
Vermiglio, F., and others. 1990. "Defective Neuromotor and Cognitive Ability in
    Iodine-Deficient Schoolchildren in an Endemic Goiter Region in Sicily." *Journal
    of Endocrinological Metabolism* 70: 379–84.
WHO (World Health Organization). 1990. "Informal Consultation on Intestinal
    Helminth Infections." Geneva.
World Bank. 1991. "Feeding Latin America's Children: An Analytical Survey of
    Food Programs." LAC Report 95-62. World Bank, Latin America and the
    Caribbean Technical Department, Human Resources Division, Washington,
    D.C.
————. 1992. "Honduras Social Investment Fund." Staff Appraisal Report.
    Washington, D.C. Available from World Bank Public Information Center,
    Washington, D.C.
————. 1994. *Enriching Lives: Overcoming Vitamin and Mineral Malnutrition in
    Developing Countries.* Washington, D.C.
Yan-you and Shu-hua. 1985. "Improvement in Hearing among Otherwise Normal
    School Children in Iodine-Deficient Areas of Guizhou China Following Use
    of Iodized Salt." *Lancet* 8454: 518–20.

Directions in Development

Begun in 1994, this series contains short essays, written for a general audience, often to summarize published or forthcoming books or to highlight current development issues.

Africa's Management in the 1990s and Beyond: Reconciling Indigenous and Transplanted Institutions

Building Human Capital for Better Lives

Class Action: Improving School Performance in the Developing World through Better Health and Nutrition

Deep Crises and Reform: What Have We Learned?

Early Child Development: Investing in the Future

Financing Health Care in Sub-Saharan Africa through User Fees and Insurance

Global Capital Supply and Demand: Is There Enough to Go Around?

Implementing Projects for the Poor: What Has Been Learned?

Improving Early Childhood Development: An Integrated Program for the Philippines

India's Family Welfare Program: Moving to a Reproductive and Child Health Approach (with a separate supplement)

Investing in People: The World Bank in Action

Managing Commodity Booms — and Busts

Meeting the Infrastructure Challenge in Latin America and the Caribbean

Monitoring the Learning Outcomes of Education Systems

MIGA: The First Five Years and Future Challenges

Nurturing Development: Aid and Cooperation in Today's Changing World

Nutrition in Zimbabwe: An Update

(continued on the following page)

Directions in Development (*continued*)